CLIMATE CHANGE
for the novice

Dike N Kalu

The opinions expressed in this book are solely the opinions of the author and do not represent the opinions or thoughts of the publisher. The author has the full ownership and legal right to publish all the materials in his book.

Dedication
This book is dedicated to my wife Carolyn, our children Nneji, Ngozi, Ndukwe and their spouses, and to all my adorable grandchildren and Nde NdukwoNta Royal Family of Abiriba.

Acknowledgements
I thank Eme N Kalu and ND Kalu for reading parts of this book and making many useful suggestions, but I retain full responsibility for any defects in the book. I also thank all the faceless and dedicated people that have made the Internet such an invaluable information resource for the discerning public.

Also, by Dike N Kalu:
Agony of a Nigerian Scientist
Science and Technology in Nigeria
Nigeria's Adventures in Technology
Climate Change for the novice + Nigeria's predicament

Contents

Preface

Climate Change is the most important event that impacts planet earth in our time because of its potential to alter life as we now know it. Interest in the subject of climate change was enhanced when the former Vice President of America, Al Gore shared the Nobel Peace Prize with the United Nations Intergovernmental Panel on Climate Change (IPCC) in 2007, for drawing the attention of the world to climate change and for laying "the foundations for the measures that are needed to counteract such change". Climate change is so important to the entire world that if it is not adequately addressed now or shortly you or your progeny will be impacted by its deleterious consequences. It is therefore essential for every individual to be knowledgeable about the basics of climate change. This is more so in the developing countries where awareness about climate change is limited because the subject has not received the magnitude of attention it deserves.

Professor Dike has summarized in this concise and easy to understand slim book all the relevant information that a novice requires to appreciate the climate change phenomenon. The original version of this book was published in 2016 and it has been abridged in 2018 to facilitate its use. This abridged version makes the book a uniquely invaluable resource for students, and all persons especially in the developing world who are interested in learning about this important emerging field of climate change.

Chapter One

Global warming/climate change

The earth's temperature is the balance between the energy entering and leaving it. The main source of energy for the earth is sunlight. Incoming energy from the sun's rays is in the form of short wavelength radiation. It enters the earth's atmosphere from the sun and reaches the surface of the earth. Some of it is reflected to space and some is absorbed, transformed into heat and warms the earth and its oceans.

With time the earth releases some of the energy it absorbed from the sun not as visible light, but as long wavelength infrared radiation or heat and the latter further heats up the lower atmosphere of the earth. Some of the infrared radiation is absorbed by *greenhouse gases (vide infra)* in the earth's atmosphere. Since these gases as it were capture and retain hot radiation from the earth, the latter is further heated up, and consequently more than the sun's radiation alone would have.

Global Warming: The earth has been warming at an accelerated rate lately. In fact, there has been an increase of about 1.4-degree Fahrenheit (0.8 degrees Centigrade) in atmospheric temperature since 1880 and a small but significant increase in temperature in all the earth's continents since the beginning of the twentieth century.

Why should one be concerned that planet earth is getting warmer?

A simple short answer is that if the temperature of the planet continues to rise unchecked, this will cause changes in the earth's climate with deleterious consequences that will make life on planet earth as we currently know it to be no longer possible. More specifically there are two intertwined potential outcomes of increased atmospheric temperatures over extended periods that are of concern: one is the difficulties and destructions that will come because of the inevitable climate change that will follow. The other concern is embodied in the following consideration:

The state of the world we live in today is the result of man's efforts to tame his environment and come to terms with it, and this has been going on for thousands of years. The gains and advances that society has made so far took into considerations the climate of planet earth. If the current rising temperatures that are occurring all over the world persist and alter the world's climate permanently the consequences will threaten the very essence of humanity and human civilization and how we live today will become history. The climate change phenomenon is complex and requires that we first touch briefly on the following to facilitate our understanding.

Weather: The degree of warmth of the earth's atmosphere is intimately related to weather and climate which are important characteristics of any environment. The weather is the condition of the atmosphere over a region for a short period of time; it could change within minutes to months. Weather includes such phenomena as temperature, humidity, precipitation, fog, sunshine, cloudiness, wind velocity, snow, storms, flooding, blizzards, cold front, warm front, etc. These conditions are taken into consideration when forecasters tell us what the weather would likely be.

Climate on the other hand is the average pattern of the weather. It is determined statistically by measuring such weather indices as temperature, humidity, wind patterns atmospheric pressure precipitation etc. over a long period of at least 30 years. This definition of climate was okay until it was found that the climate of a place did not persist unchanged for such a long time and that significant changes could be evident within a decade. While weather may persist for only a short time, the climate of a region can last for hundreds to thousands and even millions of years.

Climate change is a variation in the climate of a region. It could be an above or below normal change in any indices of weather such as temperature lasting for decades or longer.

While global warming is prolonged elevated average temperature of the globe, climate change refers to a change in the climate of a region in the globe. Climate change typically occurs because of a prolonged change in the average temperature, but strictly speaking climate change does not mean global warming.

Sustained high environmental temperature can cause heat waves leading to deadly diseases like heat cramp and stroke. It can also affect the oceans which gradually absorb the heat, cause coastal storms, alter weather patterns, increase melting of snow and ice in the polar regions, and it can trigger other changes in the indices of climate as we are currently seeing in different parts of the world.

These changes in climate include the frequent occurrence of heavy rainfalls, excessive hot weather, droughts, rising sea levels, flooding, altered onset and length of seasons, altered melting of ice in the Arctic and Antarctic regions and the shrinking of mountain glaciers. The above evidence of changes in the climate is like the result of a prolonged increased warming of the earth. Therefore, climate change has rightly been described by some as the consequence of global warming. Since the outcomes of global warming and climate change are basically the same, in certain quarters both terms are used interchangeably. However, many people prefer to use climate change for either term because climate change more readily draws attention to other changes that might occur because of the warming of the globe. In fact, these other changes such as floods, hurricanes, storms, cyclones and tornadoes may even have greater destructive impact on human lives than a sole increase in global temperature. In this text we consider *climate change* and *global warming* to be both interchangeable and virtually the same.

Education and climate change: One of the obstacles to appreciating the climate change phenomenon amongst the masses in undereducated societies is the burden of illiteracy. In addition to other things, illiteracy results in a lack of awareness of the interrelationships between the environment and factors like energy, the climate, geologic activities, the oceans, and the ice-caps in the polar regions.

Education informs us that the earth rotates in its orbit around the sun which is the source of the earth's heat and energy. A slight change in the earth's orbit will result in a change in the amount of sun's energy the earth receives, and consequently this might change the earth's temperature. Volcanoes due to geologic events can increase the levels of atmospheric greenhouse gases *(vide infra)* that absorb heat and increase the earth's temperature, or they could release into the atmosphere particles and aerosols that reflect sunlight away from the earth and so cool our globe.

Also, education reinforces the fact that the temperatures of the earth is not static but can change depending on circumstances. In the past the earth's temperature varied enormously over time. For instance, fossil plants and the remains of extinct large herbivorous dinosaurs suggest that over 100 million years ago, the Antarctica region supported a subtropical condition and not the polar ice cap that we see today. Scientists have determined that during that period the climate of the earth was about 5-8 degrees Centigrade warmer than it is today.

Also, relevant to this discussion is the fact that education informs us that the earth has in the past endured four ice ages with very cold atmospheric temperatures. These ice ages were separated by interglacial periods with slightly warmer temperatures. That these facts are not common knowledge especially in developing countries high-lights the necessity to strengthen the type of education that is relevant for this age of climate change.

In summary to appreciate the climate change phenomenon education is paramount. One needs to understand that the earth's temperature can warm or cool when the amount of solar energy reaching it alters because of the addition of *forcing* into the atmosphere.

Climate forcing is an external factor that when added into the atmosphere makes the earth's climate to change. Forcings occur naturally on earth as greenhouse gases (*vide infra*) and they are also released during volcanic activities to the atmosphere where they can warm or cool the earth. These we know and accept. It was only when the cause of the warming of the earth was associated with the introduction of forcings into the earth's atmosphere through man's activities that the subject of global warming/climate change began to attract vociferous skeptics and deniers *(vide infra)*.

Chapter Two

Causes of global warming climate change

The cause(s) of the recent rapid increase in global temperature was for a long time enigmatic and later it became a source of acrimonious debates.

Natural causes: Since it is the energy from the sun that normally makes the earth's temperature warm, it is logical to enquire whether the current increase in global temperature associated with climate change originated directly from the sun. In fact, changes in the earth's climate in the past were attributable to *natural* variations in solar radiation of the earth. These variations occurred because of small changes in the earth's orbit or because of release into the atmosphere of volcanic particles that absorb heat or reflect sunlight's rays away from the earth as discussed earlier. However according to a British geological survey "the contribution to the present-day atmospheric CO2 loading *(major cause of global warming)* from volcanic emissions------ is relatively insignificant". In addition, satellite data from the 1970s show no indication of upward trend in the amount of energy reaching the earth from the sun as a slight change in orbit would indicate. Moreover, from 1950 to 2005 the sun was relatively less active and yet atmospheric temperature kept rising. These observations indicate that it is unlikely that the recent progressive warming of the earth is due to natural causes related to the sun.

Human Causes: Climate change is *not a theory*. It has occurred before as is beautifully illustrated by the finding that despite its present polar ice covering, the Antarctica previously supported subtropical conditions with much higher temperatures than today's.

During the industrial revolution which began around 1760 in England and gradually spread to other countries, people started to turn from home and hand-based production of goods to methods that involved large-scale manufacturing. As the industrial revolution proceeded, manufacturing quickly became a staple in the evolution of human "civilization". Fossil fuels were introduced to meet the resultant energy needs for large-scale manufacturing in factories. The burning of fossil fuels led to the production of greenhouse gases which grab heat from infrared radiation from the earth's surface and so make the earth warmer. Therefore, unbeknown to the public the industrial revolution resulted in the continuous pouring into the earth's atmosphere of greenhouse gases *(vide infra)* which progressively increased the earth's temperature and eventually caused global warming and climate change.

The skeptics and deniers: While most people in Europe and around the world agree with the above scenario, many in the USA are still not fully aligned with the tenets of climate change phenomenon. Notable among these were the skeptics and deniers who impeded and frustrated advances in the understanding of global warming by constantly finding faults with any evidence that supported climate change including its being man-made. These deniers tried at all cost to cast doubt in the minds of the public about the validity of climate change.

Climate change is a scientific issue, and science is adversarial in nature. So, there is nothing wrong with disagreements among scientists about any aspect of an emerging scientific field as such disagreements usually lead to more scrutiny and enquiry. Eventually, based on the available facts a consensus is arrived at that leads to a better understanding of the issue in question. However, it seemed that the few vocal individuals that resisted global warming/climate change had a different agenda besides just seeking for a better scientific understanding of the emerging field.

These skeptics and deniers appeared to be knowingly bent on delaying the emergence of the new discipline of climate change. They raised unwarranted doubts about all aspects of climate change: its human causation, the nature of its deleterious consequences and its impacts on society, and by so doing they fanned the fears of those who were primarily concerned about the economic consequences of climate change. The deniers were concerned that acknowledging man's role in causing global warming will legitimize the large demands liberals would make to control it and its devastating consequences.

Many dissenters that continued to frustrate legitimate mainstream scientific views about climate change were outright deniers; some posed as scientific skeptics who seemed to be only concerned about seeking the truth about climate change. However eventually it became known that the agenda of the so-called skeptics were virtually the same as those of the deniers. The conspiracy of the skeptics and deniers was further blown when investigative journalism revealed that all along oil companies were aware that burning oil and gas for energy production could cause the climate to change. The financial supporters of the deniers were mostly conservative donors and oil companies who have vested financial interest in the lack of public acceptance or even delay in the emergence of climate change as a legitimate phenomenon.

Fortunately, or unfortunately politics also entered the fray of climate change controversy. Conservative republicans denied the existence of man-made global warming, and under their administration funding for climate warming-related issues was drastically curtailed or stopped. In contrast, Al Gore then a young congressman and Democrat aligned himself with top scientists studying climate change and he championed global warming campaign in Congress. Later he wrote the book "An Inconvenient Truth" which became a best seller and was turned into a movie. In 2007 he and the United Nations' body IPCC were jointly awarded the Nobel Peace Prize for laying the "foundations for the measures that are needed to counteract" climate change. The IPCC (UNs Intergovernmental Panel on Climate Change) merits additional "thank you" for their perseverance and leadership in doing the necessary scientific spade work in Climate Change.

The silver lining in the climate change controversy is that partly because of the objections of skeptics and deniers, proponents examined exhaustively the possible causes of climate change. Their results always matched their previous conclusions: Natural factors do not play a significant role in the recent, marked, progressive increase in global temperature; rather greenhouse effect due to the burning of fossil fuels by man is the principal culprit. Scientists have now closed their books on the global warming/climate change controversy, and rightly so.

Chapter Three

Greenhouse effect

Gases and atmospheric temperatures: Scientists have determined that small amounts of some naturally occurring gases in the atmosphere play a big role in maintaining the temperature of the earth at the livable level of about 15 degrees Centigrade. Without these gases the temperature of the earth would have been a very low frigid -18 degrees Centigrade. The gases are called greenhouse gases (GHGs) because the mechanism by which they elevate the earth's temperature can be likened to how high temperatures are achieved in a greenhouse.

A greenhouse is not a green-painted enclosure; rather it is an enclosed dome or building made see-through with glass or plastic. Greenhouses are used as production facilities for green vegetables and flowers that require high temperatures to grow. A greenhouse absorbs short wavelength radiation from the sun's rays through glass or plastic and thereby heats the inside of the enclosure. The heat produces long wavelength radiation which remains inside the enclosure and makes it warmer. As more heat is retained in the greenhouse than goes out, the temperature inside builds up and with time it gets very hot as in a car left outside on a sunny hot day.

In a similar manner greenhouse gases occurring naturally in the earth's atmosphere allow short wavelength radiation from the sun's rays to enter the earth's lower atmosphere unimpeded. The sun's rays heat the earth's surface and lead to the generation of long wavelength infrared heat energy that is radiated into the atmosphere. This heat is captured by the naturally occurring greenhouse gases and warms the earth.

If there were no natural greenhouse gases in the earth's atmosphere any heat emitted by the earth would just pass the earth's atmosphere and get lost to space. However, because of the presence of natural though small levels of greenhouse gases in the atmosphere these gases trap the heat radiated from the earth and thereby keep atmospheric temperature higher than if the sun was the only source of the earth's warming. This is the *greenhouse effect* which is believed to have been occurring for millions of years to keep the earth warm. This being so, it is reasonable to assume that if the amount of greenhouse gases in the earth's atmosphere increases, more heat will be trapped by these gases and the earth's atmosphere will become correspondingly warmer. This is exactly what the global warming proponents say. They hold the view that in our planet today, there are two components to greenhouse effect. The first component is the result of a small amount of GHGs found naturally in the earth's atmosphere, and the second is the result of large amounts of GHGs that are being added to the atmosphere daily because of burning fossil fuels for energy by man. These greenhouse gases generated by man, are proposed to be the main cause of global warming /climate change.

Which are the greenhouse gases? The GHGs include carbon dioxide, methane, nitrous oxide, water vapor, ozone and chlorofluorocarbons (CFCs). The GHGs are positive forcings that push the climate system in the direction of warming. Although water vapor can also capture heat and increase atmospheric temperature many consider its importance, as you will see later, to reside more on it having positive feedback effect on heat generated by other GHGs.

The importance of a GHG depends on its atmospheric concentration, its lifetime in the atmosphere, and its global warming potential (GWP). The latter is the amount of heat a gas traps in the atmosphere compared to the amount trapped by carbon dioxide (CO2) under identical conditions. To facilitate comparisons, the GWP of CO2 is set at 1 and other gasses are assigned numbers compared with the value for CO2. A brief description of the individual GHGs follows.

Carbon Dioxide is the primary greenhouse gas. It is present naturally in the atmosphere as part of the earth's carbon cycle in which carbon circulates among the atmosphere, oceans, soil, plants and animals. As I alluded to previously, carbon dioxide and other GHGs have been increasing in the atmosphere since the industrial revolution because of the burning of fossil fuels for energy by man.

Man did not only introduce excessive amounts of CO_2 into the atmosphere, he also interferes with the natural process for removing CO_2 from the atmosphere. He does this by altering the way he utilizes and manages the land in his environment. Since prehistoric times man has influenced how he uses land in his environment because land is necessary for social and economic reasons. After man discovered agriculture, he began to clear large areas for farming, and he started to build cities and towns and engage in other developmental activities. These undertakings were associated with deforestation. Clearing and using the land for farming, housing, agriculture and other economic developments is *land use change*. This change in how man used the land before the industrial revolution did not occur without costs. *Land use change* increased the temperature of the environment. This occurs as follows: Plants absorb, use and store CO_2 as they grow and mature. The soil also stores a large amount of CO_2 and it is home to numerous carbon-based microorganisms. The storage of CO_2 by forest trees, plants and the soil is known as *biological carbon sequestration*. Since this process takes CO_2, a major greenhouse gas out of the atmosphere, forest trees and pants are also called *greenhouse sinks*.

When trees are cut down to create space for agriculture, urban buildings or development, the natural sink for CO_2

is removed as the tree trunks and dead leaves can no longer absorb and hold CO2. Consequently, CO2 accumulates in the atmosphere. If the deforestation is followed by the tilling of the ground as in farming there is a further increase in the release of CO2 from the soil into the atmosphere. Tilled grounds often turn into grasslands, and like agricultural plants or trees sometimes planted to replace forest trees, they have less capacity for storing CO2 than forest trees. Since about 50% of the dry weight of wood is carbon, burning forest trees or leaving them to rot further increases atmospheric CO2 as stored carbon is released into environment. If wood from the forest is turned into lumber for sell, carbon dioxide remains locked in the wood. However, the net effect of clearing trees and forests is an increase in atmospheric CO2.

Deforestation alone has been estimated to contribute about 23% of current man-made CO2 emissions. The net effect of these increased levels of CO2 is increase in atmospheric temperature because of the ability of CO2 to capture heat derived from the sun rays. So, *land use change* by increasing environmental temperature contributes to global warming and climate change.

A small amount of CO2 is also released into the atmosphere as a byproduct during the manufacture of cement.

Methane is the second most important greenhouse gas. It is estimated that over 60% of atmospheric methane come from human activities and that its concentration in the air has doubled since the industrial revolution. Humans contribute to methane emissions mainly through their activities in industry, agriculture and waste management.

Methane is the main component of natural gas used commonly as fuel source. It is released while being obtained from underground sources for industrial purposes and from leaky fuel pipes while pumping oil and mining coal. Natural sources of methane include wetlands, decomposing organic wastes in nature, garbage dumps and bacteria that decompose organic materials anaerobically. Rice cultivation and enteric fermentation in farm animals are big sources of atmospheric methane. Large quantities of methane are present in ice crystals as clathrate deposits at the bottom of sea beds and in deep permafrost of frozen plants and animals. Clathrates and permafrost are potential big contributors to atmospheric methane when environmental temperature gets warm. In addition to being a greenhouse gas in its own right, methane may be gradually converted to carbon dioxide while it is in the atmosphere.

Methane's global warming potential (GWP) is about 20 times that of carbon dioxide but its lifetime in the atmosphere is only 12 years, much shorter than that of carbon dioxide which can remain in the atmosphere for a thousand or more years.

Nitrous oxide: Nitrous oxide is naturally present as a component of nitrogen cycle in plants, animals and microorganisms in soil and water from where it is emitted into the atmosphere. Nitrous oxide is emitted when transportation fuels are burned and as a byproduct in industrial activities such as production of nitric acid, nylons and other synthetic products. Nitrogen-rich fertilizers which are used liberally by farmers in agriculture are major contributors to atmospheric nitrous oxide. The latter is used in dentistry (laughing gas) to relieve pain and anxiety, and as a favorite oxidizer in rocket motors.

Nitrous oxide makes a much smaller contribution to atmospheric GHGs than methane. This is because its concentration in the atmosphere is small in comparison to that of methane. Nevertheless, nitrous oxide is a significant GHG for many reasons: it is a powerful heat capturing agent with a GWP of 297 in comparison to a GWP of 20 for methane and 1 for CO_2; its lifetime in the atmosphere is about 120 years, ten times more than that of methane.

Water vapor is the most dominant greenhouse gas, and it is estimated to account for about 60% of the heating effect of greenhouse gases. It is particularly important because it also amplifies existing temperature and the warming effect of other greenhouse gases. Water vapor cannot be added to the earth's atmosphere as other forcings can. But it can hold heat derived from the forcings and thereby make the environment warmer. This is how it works: The amount of water vapor in the atmosphere is determined by atmospheric temperature. If a forcing like CO2 is added to the atmosphere the temperature increases because CO2 being a greenhouse gas captures heat. The increased temperature causes water to evaporate from land and oceans and thereby increases water vapor concentration in the atmosphere. Water vapor being a greenhouse gas absorbs thermal energy and causes a further increase in atmospheric temperature; the latter again increases the heating of the land and oceans which leads to further increase in atmospheric temperature. This process in which an increase in atmospheric temperature leads to further increase in temperature is known as *positive feedback,* and it is the main mechanism by which water vapor increases atmospheric temperature. Water vapor will exert this positive feedback effect no matter which greenhouse gas caused the initial increase in atmospheric temperature; hence its dominance as a greenhouse gas.

Adding more water vapor to the atmosphere through the above positive feedback can lead to more cloud formation. As evaporation from land and ocean continues the cloud thickens as it is laden with water. When the cloud is saturated, rainfall ensues following a slight drop in the temperature. So, unlike the other GHGs water vapor is *condensable* into cloud which will remain only a short time in the atmosphere and then dissipates as rain. This is unlike other forcings that remain in the atmosphere for a very long time.

The greenhouse effect of water vapor explains why a cloudy day is much warmer than a day without clouds as illustrated by the following scenario: During the day atmospheric temperature was found to be 32 degrees Centigrade (89.6 degrees F), and the sky was covered by a blanket of cloud filled with water vapor. In the night you could not sleep because the temperature remained hot, but in another day, you were able to sleep even though the day temperature was also 32 degrees Centigrade. *Why? Answer:* The high day temperature of the first day warmed the earth and increased the temperature of the atmosphere which in turn increased atmospheric water vapor. Water vapor in cloud being a greenhouse gas absorbed the heat in the atmosphere and prevented it from escaping, making the night to remain unbearably hot as during the day.

In another occasion, although the day temperature was again 32 degrees Centigrade, as the water vapor thickened rain ensued. The water vapor and cloud were washed out by rain, and the sky became clear and blue. You enjoyed your sleep at night because the atmospheric temperature had fallen appreciably, and the night was cool. This is because although the sun had warmed the earth to 32 degrees Centigrade during the day, there was no water vapor in the sky to absorb the heat which then escaped into space and left the lower atmosphere cool.

Cloud also has the capacity to reflect light energy coming from the sun's rays back into space thereby lowering temperature and cooling the earth through *negative feedback*. So, the effect of water vapor/cloud on atmospheric temperature is quite complex and still under active study.

Ozone and the F gases: Ozone is constantly produced and destroyed naturally at about 19 – 30 km above the earth's surface. There it forms the ozone layer which filters out UV rays from the sun and thereby protects the earth from the deleterious consequences of the sun's UV radiation such as sunburn which can lead to skin cancer. Although damage to the ozone layer can expose the earth's surface to the sun's rays, UV radiation from the sun is not believed to be the cause of the current warming of the earth's atmosphere.

While ozone can capture heat from the atmosphere, it is difficult to quantify its contribution to global warming because it is present in the earth's atmosphere in small quantities. It lasts in the atmosphere for only a few days or weeks, and its concentration around the world is not uniform but varies markedly from region to region.

Other chemicals that can capture heat and increase the temperature of the globe are the F-gases, namely: chlorofluorocarbons (CFCs), hydrochlorofluorocarbons (HCFCs), perfluorocarbons (PFCs) and sulfur hexafluoride (SF6). These chemicals are man-made for various commercial purposes, and their concentrations in the atmosphere are small. However, they have long lifetimes and high heat-capturing capacities and their emissions can potentially influence the climate for decades or even centuries. Because they can also destroy the ozone layer, their production is regulated by international agreements and many of them have been banned and are no longer produced in industrialized nations.

Chapter Four

Impacts of climate change

As I have indicated before climate change is currently occurring worldwide in different places at varying degrees. Its impacts are manifest as the recent extremes of weather that various parts of the world are experiencing such as melting of ice caps in the tundra regions, scorching temperatures, incessant heavy rains, swollen oceans and seas, frequent heavy floods and erosions, altered seasons, disrupted agriculture, poor farming yields, starvation, etc.

So, changes in the climate have deleterious consequences on ecosystems on land and in oceans, transportation, water supplies, people's homes, agriculture, livelihood and even human health. The prediction is that these negative impacts will get worse if nothing substantive is done about climate change, and life on earth as we know it will have to change and at a great cost. This should be of concern to all for at least one reason: human civilization and the present state of the world irrespective of its imperfections are the result of the evolution of society that has occurred over thousands of years; that this state is now under threat of obliteration by climate change is real.

Basis of the effects of climate change: Any of the individual effect of climate change can be traced back to an initial progressive rise in atmospheric temperature. The impact climate change has on people varies according to what part of the world they reside in and the exact location of their dwelling. For instance, the effect of climate change on people that live in arid areas of the world and far inland will be different from its impact on those people that live near coasts or near ice and glaciers in the poles. Climate change impacts call for being particularly sensitive to what is happening to water levels because 70% of the globe is covered by water. The level of sea water (which is basically that part of the ocean that is nearest to land) rises when elevated environmental temperature causes ice and snow to melt and the water is delivered into the ocean. High temperatures will also cause water to expand and enlarge its volume thereby augmenting a rise in sea level and enhancing susceptibility to floods due to elevated atmospheric temperature.

In general, persistently high atmospheric temperature or global warming/climate change as is occurring on planet earth now will make wet places wetter and dry places drier. Elevated temperature will increase evaporation of water from land, sea and ocean and this will in turn increase the amount of atmospheric water vapor. If this continues, the upper atmosphere becomes saturated with water-laden clouds which eventually results in rain as previously described. In climate change situations this occurs frequently and heavily because of persistently high atmospheric temperatures. The rain could be accompanied by floods, storms and hurricanes which would cause even more disastrous effects than elevated temperature alone in the areas concerned.

Since climate change occurs world-wide its impacts will also be seen in arid and semi-arid regions. The people that reside in these areas of the world are some of the poorest of the poor, and their world is characterized by extremely high temperatures, water scarcity and low productivity of the land leading to food scarcity, hunger and short life expectancy. Migration to the cities in search of food is common practice in these areas. The high temperature of climate change by causing the already high local temperature to be even higher and more erratic, exacerbates the dry, harsh conditions in arid and semi-arid regions and makes life more intolerable for the unfortunate inhabitants of these arid/semi-arid regions of the world.

One need not aim at being able to recite all the known deleterious consequences of climate change and where they have occurred. What will be more useful is to be able to anticipate the possible disastrous consequences of prolonged excessive atmospheric temperature on your environment and figuring out beforehand how to mitigate against such a disastrous outcome.

European Union Commission findings: For more information on the impacts of climate change around the world, the United Nation's Intergovernmental Panel on Climate Change (IPCC) is an invaluable resource. It cannot be overstated that if left unchecked the effects of climate change and their possible impacts on humans and their environments will be disastrous beyond our imagination. The European Commission which is the executive body of the European Union (EU) also had a grim assessment of the consequences of climate change. I have itemized below a summary of their findings and conclusions from a recent survey of the issue.

Regions evaluated	Consequences of climate change
1. Southern and Central Europe	More frequent heat waves and forest fires
2. Mediterranean area	Drier, more vulnerable to droughts and fire
3. Northern Europe	Wetter, winter floods may become more common
4. Urban areas	Susceptible to heat waves, flooding or rising sea levels. Inhabitants are often ill-equipped to adapt to climate change
5. Developing countries	Depend heavily on their natural environment for sustenance. Have the least resources to cope with changing climate

6. Risk for Human health	Increase in the number of heart related deaths in some regions and a decrease in cold related deaths in others
7. Cost for economy and society	Damage to property, infrastructure and human health. Sectors affected most are those that rely more on certain temperatures and precipitation levels such as agriculture, forestry and energy and tourism.
8. Risks for wild life	Many plants and animal species are struggling to cope. Many terrestrial, freshwater and marine species have already moved to new locations. Some plant and animal species will be at risk of extinction if global temperatures continue to rise unchecked

Chapter Five

Climate change in Developing countries

Athough developing countries did not participate in the industrial revolution that initiated climate change nor share in the immediate economic fallouts and benefits from it, they and other people around the world are feeling its projected deleterious impacts. These impacts of climate change are not uniform in all places and do not come with a stamp of identity or origin. As a result, some in the developing world see them as just another of those unwholesome difficulties that periodically visit them and that they are incapable of handling without foreign assistance. Nothing could be farther from the truth.

Nigerian Environmental Study Team (NEST): In 1987, a year before the United Nations formed the now august body, Intergovernmental Panel on Climate Change (IPCC), the Nigerian Environmental Study Team (NEST) was established as a non-governmental organization (NGO) under the able leadership of Professor David Okali (Emeritus) of Ibadan University. Since then NEST has been doing ground-breaking work on threats to the Nigerian environment including the detrimental impacts of climate change.

To examine the far-reaching effects of climate change which originated from energy use by Europeans in the 18th century, let us briefly consider the plight of a farmer today in the developing African country called Nigeria. In the 18th century Nigeria was not in existence and surely the indigenes of the area now called Nigeria played no role in making fossil fuels the preferred energy source of the world. In one lecture on *Climate Change* Professor Okali of NEST showed a cartoon of an illiterate Nigerian farmer that had an inexplicable turn of events with the source of his livelihood. This individual was previously a very successful and prosperous farmer, but lately he could no longer ply his trade profitably because the seasons had become terribly disrupted and unfavorable for farming. Droughts had become commonplace and had been lasting longer than living memory could remember. When it rained it was unimaginably heavy and long; the planting season had disappeared; if a farmer dared to plant notwithstanding, the harvest was pathetic. For the first time in a long time even farmers became victims of food scarcity and hunger. This was just too much for the unfortunate illiterate Nigerian farmer to bear; he could not figure out what the problem was, and eventually he took his own life by hanging. But sadly, he was not alone. He and his colleagues were not aware that they had unintentionally become the guests of climate change and its untoward consequences.

Developing nations and hostile environments: Most people in the developing world continue to wonder why the environment is recently turning very hostile. Many have witnessed and reported the environment being plagued by horrible changes such as: weather extremes, persistent erratic changes in climate, disruption of seasonal cycles, drying up of spring-sources, increased desertification in arid areas, prolonged periods of heavy rainfalls, giant erosions from rains, sand-storms that threaten living and farm lands, declines in crop yields, abnormally low marine productivity of fishermen, loss of soil fertility and agricultural productivity leading to food insecurity, damage to housing, buildings and infrastructure due to above normal wind intensity, and disruption of agriculture by long periods of droughts and heavy off-season rain-falls. Rebecca Reynolds of London School of Economics and other notables pointed out that these are all evidence of the untoward consequences of climate change. When climate change disaster impacts you in an obvious way, it is already late to be able to manage it and you will be forced to pay a big price. Therefore, the work of United Nations' IPCC and indigenous nongovernmental groups like Nigeria's NEST is so commendable and worthy of support, and people should act now.

Rebecca Reynolds also emphasized that both *developed* and *developing countries* are equally susceptible to the damaging impacts of global change. She reminded us that all over the world poor people will be more vulnerable to the disastrous effects of climate change than the well-off. Since poverty is more rampart in developing countries, she argued that the latter are therefore more susceptible to the deleterious consequences of climate change than developed nations.

Developing countries are particularly prone to the deleterious consequences of climate change for many reasons: First, developing countries depend heavily on their natural environment for sustenance and therefore will be greatly impacted by a disturbance of the environment in the scale that climate change will generate. Second, the poor in developing countries live in substandard unplanned dwellings in areas more prone to storm surges and flooding. They are economically disadvantaged and do not have infrastructural and technological capacity and resources to adequately respond to such natural disasters as are associated with climate change. Third, in developing countries awareness among the people of the true nature of the impending problems that will come with climate change is scant. The reasons for this lie squarely on the shoulders of developing countries' governments whose duty it is to eradicate illiteracy and promote awareness. Fourth, most developing countries already have plateful of other national and humanitarian problems confronting them, and climate change disaster will just have to take its place in terms of priority.

Chapter Six

What can be done about climate change?

Global challenge: Climate change is a complex global problem and ideally it requires the entire global community to mount an effective unified strategy to counter it and its adverse effects. A combat strategy that will be acceptable to all nations is complicated by many factors. Most notably is the fact that climate change transverses many important areas such as science, technology, economics, politics, ethics, literacy and the entire industrialized and developing countries with their differing circumstances and priorities.

A realistic plan to fight climate change must, also consider the special plight of developing countries who have argued that the industrialized nations should bear the responsibility for cleaning up the untoward effects of climate change because they caused it. Many believe the developed nations are culpable because they introduced excessive amounts of GHGs into the world's atmosphere and have had the lion's share of the benefits for ushering in climate change through their continued use of fossil fuels as their energy source. To ameliorate climate change and its damaging effects a plea has been made to limit or abandon the use of fossil fuels. In response, developing countries have argued that it is unfair to ask them to stop doing what industrialized countries have already done to develop their own countries. It is unjust, they say to ask them to stop using convenient, easily available fossil fuels and lumber from deforestation to build their infrastructure and economy as the industrialized countries have already done.

If climate change is not addressed soon and the anticipated associated calamities befall the entire earth, the advanced nations will naturally look after their own citizens first before worrying about the developing countries. Therefore, every developing country should invest in a Climate Change Disaster Program (no matter how modest) that focuses on those areas in their local environments that are likely to be vulnerable to the deleterious effects of climate change. Such a program in developing countries should also invest substantively on regular and adult education efforts that raise the awareness of all citizens to the reality of climate change issues. Nonetheless, the two main approaches available world-wide for addressing climate change are adaptation and mitigation.

Adaptation is developing ways to protect people and the environment from existent and projected adverse consequences of climate change. In other words, in adaptation man still lives with climate change, its causes and deleterious consequences but he figures out ways to circumvent the adverse effects. For instance, he stops building his dwellings on the coast to avoid being washed away by the inevitable floods that will come because of heavy rains and rise in sea level due to climate change. The emphasis here is on managing the possible adverse consequence of climate change.

Even before reaching an effective global management agreement for climate change, many governments and communities in several parts of the world started using adaptive measures to protect their people. This is because of the enormity of the adverse consequences of climate change which, as previously pointed out, are already occurring in many places around the world.

Adaptive measures for climate change that people often consider include: building sea walls to protect citizens against rising sea levels and floods; moving dwellings away from coastal areas; diversifying crop varieties to include those that are more tolerant to heat, drought and waterlogging; protecting livestock from hot temperatures; increasing energy efficiency of appliances, etc. In fact, in adaptation society adjusts in any way feasible to overcome or minimize the negative impacts of climate change while still living with its causes.

If man were to rely only on adaptation, then he would be condemned to life-long continued struggle against the adverse consequences of climate change. What will eliminate such a perpetual struggle is to have an environment that is free of the primary cause of climate change. Therefore, an additional approach used for addressing climate change is mitigation.

Mitigation: In contrast to adaptation, mitigation involves attempts to slow the progress of climate change by eliminating from the atmosphere excessive levels of the greenhouse gases (GHGs) which are its primary cause. There are two main ways to accomplish this: one is to plant trees to serve as carbon sinks that absorb atmospheric carbon dioxide which they use for photosynthesis. In photosynthesis green plants utilize energy in sunlight to convert carbon dioxide and water to sugar and oxygen. It is worth noting that trees seem to have been quite effective in eliminating excess atmospheric CO2 from the atmosphere in pre-industrial times before man started to pour large amounts of greenhouse gases into the atmosphere by burning fossil fuels. Unfortunately, nothing was done at that time to get rid of the resultant increase in CO2 in the environment. Trees are of great benefit to our environment, and among their many functions, they have been described as the lungs of planet earth. While man breathes in oxygen and breaths out CO2, trees mop up CO2 and use it to produce oxygen and sugar which man needs.

Another way to slow climate change by mitigation is to stop putting greenhouse gases into the environment by burning fossil fuels. While it is not feasible to stop using fossil fuels "cold-turkey" in view of the reliance on fossil fuels for energy world-wide, man has started to explore ways to curb its utilization. In this regard much is being done in transportation, because transportation is the second major carbon emitter (behind electricity and before industry). Since cars are the main source of transportation-related GHG-emission, governments with automobile manufacturing economies all over the world are very interested in increasing the fuel efficiency of cars which will in turn result in a diminution in the use of fossil fuels which generate GHGs. In the US the Obama administration required the fuel efficiency of cars and light-duty trucks to average 55 miles per gallon by model year 2025, from about 36 mpg. In Europe the law targets 58 mpg for 2020 cars and later models. Progress in this area is slow because the technologies needed for success have not yet been perfected but are still being developed.

Because of need to curb the magnitude of GHG production due to transportation additional measures have been introduced by various governments and institutions to mitigate against transportation-induced increase in atmospheric GHGs. These measures include: giving people incentives to get older cars off the road in return for buying more fuel-efficient ones; tax schemes to encourage purchase of low CO2 emission cars; penalizing auto manufacturers that do not meet efficiency target for a given calendar year; giving incentives for making electric vehicles and hybrid cars that utilize less gasoline and electricity, and for inventing any technologies that will cause a real reduction in GHGs.

Individual challenge: The struggle against climate change should not just be left to the governments of various countries. While it is important for governments to show leadership and direction in the fight against climate change, we should realize that it is the citizens of the world that cause climate pollution and so we as a people are obligated to modify our individual actions and behaviors if we are serious about decreasing or even stopping climate change. Therefore, the United Nations, the Environmental Protection Agency (EPA) of America and other well-meaning organizations and individuals around the world have been advocating for individual involvement in the fight against climate change. Some have gone as far as compiling lists of things everyone should be doing to reduce atmospheric GHGs and conserve energy and thereby contribute in the fight against climate change. Highest in most lists is the need to limit the use of electricity which today has the greatest demand for fossil fuels.

Dos and don'ts: It is of interest that if you compare the "dos and don'ts" from different sources advocating individual involvement in the fight against climate change, you always see only two or three items that are similar, and then the rest of the items listed are different. And yet the differing items are all correct because they share the fact that directly or indirectly, they all result in the emissions of GHGs or they utilize fossil fuel-based-electricity. The existence of so many differing but correct lists shows how pervasive climate change mediators have become in our society and why everybody can and should contribute in a grassroots effort to fight against this change in our climate. Below is my compilation of ten things from different sources that individuals should be doing to help in the fight against climate change. I encourage you to make your own list and compare it with mine:

1. The car: Many people own or aim to own a car. In some cases, it is a necessity; in some it's just for pleasure, and in others it is considered a status symbol! All cars emit GHGs from the burning of fossil fuel for energy. If you must own one, buy a car that has good fuel efficiency.

2. Drive sparingly: It is not everything we do that requires driving our cars. So whenever possible don't drive; instead use public mass transit, bike or walk.

3. Air tight homes: Most homes in industrialized countries have provisions to be heated in the winter or be cooled in the summer or both. To do this you require energy which comes to a large extent from burning fossil fuels. Make your homes air tight to reduce air leaks and stop drafts; install insulation around your house and in the attic to conserve energy. Use cross-ventilation in the tropics and sub-tropical regions to reduce the need for air condition.

4. Efficient use of water: It requires a lot of energy to produce safe, clean water which should be available to everyone in any community. So, around the home conserve water by repairing toilets and leaky faucets; use your dish-washer only when it is full; do not let

water run to waste when you are shaving or brushing your teeth; water your lawn only when it is necessary, and preferably when it is cool to avoid wasteful evaporation. Public pumps should not be left running when the vessel used to collect water is full.

5. Lawn mowers and leaf blowers: Both usually run on gasoline that produce greenhouse gases, or on electricity that increases demand for fossil fuels. Whenever necessary use push mower, cutlass or machete to cut your lawn.

6. Electricity: Electricity merits special mention as it is responsible for the largest demand for burning fossil fuels for energy. The world basically runs on energy, and electric energy is used for a wide variety of purposes including to power industry and light appliances in homes and industry. Because our homes have now been invaded by apparently indispensable electrical gadgets, you should use these tools wisely. Both at home and at work use energy-saving light bulbs and appliances that are certified to last long and/or only consume little energy and switch off electric lights and computers when they are not in use.

7. Heavy home appliances: Replace your heavy electrical equipment like refrigerators, washing machines and dish washers with high efficiency, energy saving models. Whenever possible line-dry washed clothes and avoid using energy-powered drier which is an obscene consumer of electricity.

8. New homes: Roofs of new homes should henceforth be fitted with solar panels that will produce much of the energy used in the home. Old homes can also install solar panels to produce some of their domestic energy use.

9. Recycle: Buy products that are recyclable and recycle wastes from your home. This is important because in addition to conserving natural resources, recycling saves energy as industry requires more energy to fabricate products directly from raw materials than from recycled cans, glass, steel, paper, plastic bags, bottles, etc.

10. Eat less meat.

Meat and climate change. Question: Prof, your recommendation to eat less meat suggests that meat contributes to climate change. Is that correct?

Professor: Am afraid the answer is yes. Although protein in meat has an established and long history of being one of the requirements for a balanced healthy diet, eating meat is also a major contributor to climate change. To appreciate this, one must be mindful of the fact that meat production in large quantities goes through livestock farming and many processes which requires many factors that increase the production of GHGs, the major cause of global warming/climate change.

For instance, growing livestock for food requires the clearing of trees to make land available for planting pasture and crops to feed farm animals. This process of deforestation leads to the elevation of the potent greenhouse gas CO2 in the manner I described previously in Chapter 3.

In addition to elevating atmospheric greenhouse CO2 through respiration, livestock (mainly cattle) is an obligatory source of large amounts of methane, which is produced naturally during digestion in animals. As I indicated earlier methane is an important GHG with global warming potential (GWP) that is 20 times that of carbon dioxide.

Like all farmlands, the land used to produce animal feeds is depleted of its natural nutrients with time, and man then adds manure and fertilizers to the barren land to restore its fertility. This leads to an increase in the emission of nitrous oxide from synthetic fertilizers and the metabolism of nitrogen to nitrous oxide. Nitrous oxide is a potent GHG with a lifetime of about 120 years in the atmosphere and a GWP of 297.

The above considerations indicate that breeding livestock for meat leads to the production of significant amounts of GHGs. Because of the sheer number of farm animals world-wide, their breeding results in a markedly high volume of atmospheric GHGs. In fact, scientists have estimated that livestock rearing and meat consumption account for a whopping 18% of global emission of GHGs and therefore play a sizable role in climate change. This has led some to advocate abandoning eating meat and adopting vegan diets instead to give the fight against climate change a chance of achieving success.

These facts about climate change and eating meat and the potential alternative options are little known by lay people. The reason they are rarely discussed by governments is mainly because politicians do not want to be intruding in the private lives of people by telling them what type of food to eat.

Chapter Seven

Alternative energy sources

Primary source of world's energy: Fossil fuels, which are currently the primary source of the world's energy were formed from organic matter during millions of years, and they have fueled the world's economy for over a century. Because fossil fuels are being depleted, they cannot be used indefinitely as they will eventually run out. Furthermore, as we have already seen the use of fossil fuels leads to the emission of GHGs that cause global warming/climate change which can do catastrophic damage to the environment. Adverse environmental effects and finite availability are enough good reasons to seek other forms of energy in place of fossil fuels.

In addition, industrialized nations are not energy-sufficient by themselves. For instance, America supplements her energy needs by ordering oil from OPEC countries like Saudi Arabia, Kuwait, Iraq and Nigeria. Dependence on external sources of oil from other countries is not without cost. Uncertainties in oil production and price and political unrest in oil producing countries lead to oil insecurity. Furthermore, powerful countries like America may feel obliged in critical international situations to acquiesce with or to defend countries due to dependence in their oil. Availability of alternative sources of energy that is different from fossil fuels will free the advanced nations to make decisions involving oil-producing countries only by the merit of the case in question. Another source of man's energy is nuclear power.

Nuclear energy is clean, and unlike fossil fuel energy it does not produce any GHGs. However, the devastating effects of nuclear energy's radioactive by-product has led some nations to abandon or plan to abandon its use as an energy source. (*See*, Nigeria's Adventures in Technology by Dike N Kalu, Amazon.com).

Alternative energy is the third source of energy available to man. Alternative energies are environmentally non-polluting and renewable in the sense that they are basically inexhaustible and available indefinitely. Note that sometimes an energy-source may be designated as the energy itself. For instance, energy derived from burning fossil fuels may also be designated as fossil energy, and energy from nuclear power may be just called nuclear energy.

The hope of industrialized nations today is to move away completely from dependence on fossil fuels as their major energy source and to use alternative sources instead. By moving to alternative energies, the level of atmospheric GHGs would eventually decrease as would their deleterious consequences. An amusing but insightful definition of *alternative energy* is "any energy source that is alternative to fossil fuels". This tongue in cheek definition is meant to emphasize the fact that an alternative energy source must be able to address the main concerns about using fossil fuel energy. For instance, an alternative energy must come from inexhaustible natural sources unlike fossil fuels which are finite and being currently depleted. In other words, alternative energy sources should be renewable naturally. In addition, alternative energy should not harm the environment by producing such by-products as GHGs or radioactivity.

The frantic efforts that are being currently made mostly in the industrialized nations to switch to alternative energy fuels should be another wake-up call to those countries, especially developing countries like Nigeria that depend virtually on oil economy. When industrialized nations abandon fossil fuels as the world's primary energy source, as I believe they will eventually do, ill-prepared oil producing nations will not be able to claim that they did not foresee the impending economic and social disasters that would befall them. Time is highly overdue for responsible governments to give meaningful attention to the diversification of their economies because the industrialized nations have already started to augment their fossil fuel energy use with alternative energy sources whenever they can.

Examples of alternative energy include: solar energy, wind energy, biomass energy, geothermal energy, hydroelectric energy and ocean energy. I will comment briefly only on the first one.

Solar energy: Solar energy is derived from the sun's radiation and has been known and used by man since the 19th century. What has been lacking is the availability of appropriate technologies to permit adequate utilization of the sun's immense energy source which is much more than is required to meet the needs of the entire world for thousands of years. Nevertheless, solar energy technologies have been evolving and the current intensity in this evolution is fueled by the appreciation by most people now that the use of fossil fuels as the world's major energy source is the main cause of the climate change that, as we've already seen, threatens the wellbeing of planet earth.

Solar energy can be used to meet a wide range of man's energy needs including cooking, heating water, space heating, operating fans, heating swimming pools, cooling buildings and generating electricity for a wide variety of domestic, industrial and economic purposes. Because of the diverse nature of the above potential uses, several different types of technologies must be developed to enable the use of solar energy for domestic and industrial purposes. Energy from the sun or solar energy can be classified into two. The first is *passive solar energy*.

Passive solar energy is used mostly for heating or cooling living spaces. There are now solar heating technologies that enable the use of the sun's rays to directly heat swimming pool water or large volumes for industrial purposes. In addition, solar heating systems can directly heat air in solar collectors, and the heat is distributed around homes or commercial buildings as needed for space heating in cold or winter months. This direct solar heating can also be used in air conditioning in hot climates. To this end, hot air is cooled with desiccants and piped around buildings to cool them, and the desiccant is regenerated with thermal energy from the sun. Alternatively, thermal heat from solar radiation could be used to drive absorption chillers which produce chilled water for space cooling indoors.

Solar rays can also provide electricity in the conventional manner. Normally electricity production occurs in power plants with the aid of a turbine generator which transforms mechanical energy into electrical energy. For instance, burning fossil energy such as coal, oil or natural gas causes water to boil and produce steam. The latter then turns a turbine leading to the generation of electricity in the traditional way. Similarly, heat coming directly from the sun can be used to create electricity in the conventional manner if enough of it is harvested to boil water and produce steam. In practice this is done in thermal power plants that use a series of mirrors to collect and intensify the sun's rays to produce enough heat and steam to turn a turbine. The second type of energy from the sun is *active solar energy*.

Active solar energy comes from the conversion of the sun's rays directly into electricity in solar cells, and the electricity is then utilized in the normal fashion to perform a variety of functions. *A solar cell* is a small electronic device about 2-4 inches in diameter, and it can be used to produce electricity directly from the sun's radiation. A ray of light from the sun contains trillions of particles called photons that are carrying the sun's energy. When the photons hit appropriately prepared solar cells, they are converted to a flow of electrons that lead to the production of a small amount of electric current and voltage. The technology used is often referred to as photovoltaic system or just PV. The electricity that each solar cell makes is very small. So many of these cells are connected and mounted together to form a panel. So *solar cells* and *solar panels* work together to produce and direct the movement of electric current. In industrialized nations many houses are now fitted with solar panels to generate some or all their electricity.

What I have briefly summarized above is how heat and electric energies are generated from the sun to serve as clean non-polluting alternatives to fossil fuel energy. While the energy currently generated from the sun is small, many people hope that by combining energies from the different alternative sources such as the sun, water, wind, etc. the world's energy needs will eventually be met. Consequently, alternative energy generation remains an area of intensive research worldwide.

CLOSING REMARKS

It should be evident from this brief coverage that the subject of climate change is an important issue that should be of interest to everyone on planet earth. The field is broad and complex, and as I stated in the beginning, my intent here is mainly to provide a simplified introduction of this important emerging field to the novice. I hope the book will help to promote and encourage awareness of climate change especially in developing countries.